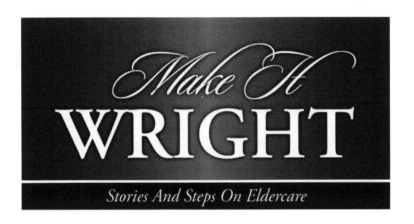

Make It WRIGHT

Stories And Steps On Eldercare

Lana A. Perry

MAKE IT WRIGHT
Stories and Steps on Eldercare

Make It Wright: Stories and Steps on Eldercare is a work of nonfiction. Persons, organizations, and events depicted in these pages are real persons and entities. All persons and stories mentioned in the text were used with permission. However, the viewpoints expressed in these stories and the lessons learned are entirely the product of the author's reflection and imagination and do not necessarily reflect the views   of any organization with which the author is affiliated. Names have been edited to protect the privacy of interviewed persons.

Entity of wrightshands publishing
www.wrightshands.com
www.wrightspublishing.com

Photography Credit: Samuel
Jordan Royal Photography LLC
www.royalphotokc.com

Book Cover Design: Shon
Burks Frozen Creative LLC
www.frozencreative.com

Editor: Patricia Perry-
Crosby Copy Editor:
Ashley Rey

Perry, Lana A. (Lana Annise), author.
   Make it Wright : stories and steps on eldercare /
by Lana A. Perry.
   pages cm
   Includes bibliographical references and
   index. ISBN 978-0-9969565-0-5

   1. Older people--Care--United States. 2.
Older people--United States--Interviews. 3.
Aging.
I. Title.

HQ1061.P344 2015   305.26
                    QBI15-1696

DEDICATION

I dedicate this work to Franzillo Wright. I prayed each day that God would take care of you on the days I couldn't provide direction or a sense of security. As each day passes, I am reminded of the wisdom you passed down to me, and the moments you shared your story with me. At the time you couldn't understand why I fought so hard to keep you away from those harming you, only to put you in another place where I couldn't protect you. It was all for God's glory. Granny, it is because of you that I am able to change the lives of others and prepare them for the elder stages of life.

ACKNOWLEDGEMENTS

To my family and friends who stuck by me when all I could do was find older adults or senior citizens to talk with. Thank you for your patience, kind words, and love. I made it my passion and promise to help elders.

To my Mom who tried her best, I say thank you. You allowed me to take over the care of Granny when you couldn't care for her yourself. From all of the teaching moments, we now have a plan for you and I can say you are aging successfully. Thank you for being open and honest, telling me what it's like, as you understand aging isn't easy. Raising a little girl who always went against the concentration gradient kept you busy. Thank you for understanding when I stepped up to care for you, it was out of love and experience. I realize accepting the role change from mother to patient and friend was not easy. Thank you to D.C., who spent hours counseling me about life and praying those long prayers. Your help in raising me *not to give up* provided me the strength to expand my vision.

To my Daddy, thank you for always believing in me and sticking by me. You pushed me into greatness, and kept on pushing me when I didn't want to follow my dreams. I learned from your love and support that no matter the family dynamic, you do what is asked of you. As your daughter, it means the world to see you fight for your life and win. For all of the daily phone calls about your health and lessons learned through your care, thank you. I will always remember Washington D.C. B.C.

To Ma Perry, I will never forget the kitchen table conversation the morning after Dad's heart surgery. In that moment, planning for the end of life helped me understand and give even more back to the community. Thank you for accepting me.

To Aunt Sharon and Uncle Rick, thank you both for your advice, help, and love. You granted me the opportunity to leave everything behind, regroup and start my life's journey. I appreciate each moment you spent listening, helping me to create the next step, and challenging my work.

To all of the people I interviewed, thank you for sharing your stories. This is your way of giving back and telling others what you wish you would've known.

This writing is for family members and friends that find themselves without direction, or in a reactive state. Caring for a loved one is never easy, and it becomes increasingly difficult when you don't have much help around you. In the early 2000's, there wasn't much literature readily available, and in one place to provide steps towards gathering information from the Office of Aging, social security, retirement, and advance care planning. I pray this book is helpful when you don't have the manpower to make 15 phone calls in order to find out what to do next in any situation. This is my story, and the stories of others who want to provide a word of encouragement, or a way to avoid pitfalls when caring for aging adults.

Contents

INTRODUCTION

As a seventeen-year-old girl, I quickly discovered that I knew nothing about aging, wisdom, or life. I did, however, understand death, but not the processes within the realm of life's end. The woman I knew and considered to be my grandmother lived 2 minutes and 38 seconds of walking distance from the front steps of my home where I grew up. From birth she was *family,* and I did not learn otherwise until my teenage years. She was the grandmother to one of my mother's students. What began as a babysitting job grew into her love for my mother as her daughter, and my sisters and me as her grandchildren.

I was introduced to aging when a good friend of Grandma's suddenly passed away. It was at this time that my grandma sat me down to explain the traumatic death of her husband and what it took to plan the ending stages of life and beyond.

Before any signs of dementia or of a deteriorating mind, Grandma planned her *own* funeral arrangements. There was tailoring the obituary, purchasing of the burial plot and headstone, choosing of the casket, and even the clothing she wanted to wear. As a seventy-nine year old woman, Grandmother progressed to a state in which she was no longer able to care to for herself. In the care of relatives who lived with her, she experienced abuse. Her home was burglarized and years of personal treasures were taken. Grandmother succumbed to a life of, practically, homelessness. On one particular Tuesday evening she was found 8 miles from her home by a stranger. He explained to me, my grandmother believed she was on her way to Sunday service at the church where we both worshipped.

One day, in Grandmother's need for help, it became very apparent and clear that only blood relatives were allowed to make life altering-decisions. A police officer devastatingly told my immediate family and I to "vacate the premises immediately" after a call was placed to authorities about her safety. Heartbroken, I turned away but saw her give me a sign through her glance that she was afraid, and still longed for help.

This is where her story only begins.

Through research, interviews and studies, I have developed practical, hands-on methods to care for aging loved ones. I hope this walkthrough will be of help to you as you ensure that your beloved elders age successfully.

Let's Bring Awareness
to the Aging Community,

One Family Member At A Time.

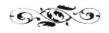

CHAPTER 1

What Is Aging?

What is aging? There is a common misconception about *what is it and how to deal with it*. According to Webster's Dictionary, aging is the process of getting older. It is not that you are old. The moment you are born, you begin the aging process. It is, what some may call, a blessing to get to an age where you have seen the world change around you.

Taking the opportunity to talk to elders is a past time that youth should partake in, because elders will share wisdom that can only come from life experiences. You have truly seen *life* when visiting friends and family has evolved to talking on a telephone and cell phone, and now to video chat. What an experience! Also take into consideration those who are of different races, religions, or cultures who may have once been persecuted for radical thinking are now seeing themselves on television or in places of power, something they probably could've never imagined. An amazing or overwhelming feeling can quickly turn into pain or depression when you experience your first senior moment. Being an older adult should be celebrated, but often times it is condemned and this can lead to elders feeling burdensome.

Patricia's Story- I'm Old

I met a woman named Patricia who is the quintessential example of the *mind changing*. She began calling herself *old* more than the usual as she approached 60. It all started at about 56 when one of her friends passed away. Her childhood friend's health began to decline, and his children decided it would be best to hire a caregiver. About six months later he passed away, and Patricia has never been the same. I sat and talked with her about death and she explained to me how she was OK with the idea because she believed God controlled her destiny. Patricia told me about her mother being killed shortly after she graduated college – a sudden change in her life - but she was able to cope.

The idea of a childhood friend dying brought on a new feeling: getting old. She felt as though life was getting shorter and her time was drawing near. She found herself feeling as if funerals were like the *new* parties. She has a collection of obituaries that almost fills half of her file drawer and relatives that she visited often were now passing away. Finally the last living aunt from her hometown was laid to rest at a church on the corner of the street where she grew up. On the day of the funeral, all of the first cousins congregated in a circle outside the small church, which made Patricia exclaim that the gatherers were now taking their parent's place. "We are getting old and we have to do better to support one another", Patricia stated.

After retiring as an educator, she made an attempt to become a substitute teacher. This new career would bring on even more challenges. Traveling to various schools and meeting others was great, but the children did not see the benefit in learning much while their teacher was absent. She felt useless, and eventually gave up the position. She, again, felt that because she was "old", it was time to sit down, and in her words "find something for old people do." Patricia is challenged in her ambulation, due to an injury that left her looking and feeling different. This in itself seems to have accelerated the feelings of "old" she experiences.

Patricia's optometrist also gave her the confirmation that she was aging. She was having difficulty seeing at night and reading books, so she scheduled an appointment. After the exam, Patricia was told that she had "old eyes". The lens of her eyes seemed *cloudy* and she was fitted with contacts, which, in turn, cosmetically, gave a brown natural look to the eyes.

In addition to experiencing cloudiness with her eyesight, she also noticed weight gain, experienced joint pain and began going to the restroom more frequently during the night. Her hair was thinning and she was forced to take vitamin supplements to combat it. She has found that the foods she once enjoyed no longer agree with her digestive track. The words "I'm old" began to get louder with each sunrise. She often reminisces about the first color TV that was sold in Sears & Roebuck, a nickel bag of chips, gas sold for 25 cents a gallon, riding the bus for a dime, and spending $10 on Christmas gifts for five different family members.

Uncontrollable physical and emotional changes ultimately lead Patricia to believe that she is *old*. The once life of ripping and running had evolved to a preference of quiet and solitude. Patricia realizes that each passing day brings her closer to a time where she may actually need help from others.

Patricia declares her patience is shorter. She loves her grandchildren, but has difficulty understanding how their parents tolerate behavior that is seemingly "disrespectful and callous". Praying most of the day, reading self–help books, listening to gospel music, and eating chocolate are her new joys in life. She feels that *what use to be* will never authentically come again, and repeated history comes, but with a "new twist."

Most importantly, she is determined to live in peace. She has taken a stance to "mind her own business" and allow others to "live their lives". She always hopes for the best, and wants to see her children make good choices. Patricia explains she does not want to be a burden on anyone, and will not ask for help because she feels as if she'll only be in the way.

The government is also constantly reminding Patricia of her age. In Ohio, you are mailed a Golden Buckeye Card to use for discounts at participating businesses and for prescription drugs. Patricia is invited to choose foods from a senior menu, and now has an AARP membership. She can't wear certain clothes anymore, and finds comfort in therapeutic footwear. Patricia's expresses that her childhood, teenage, and young adult years are gone and never to return. "I'm just old now", Patricia says.

Patricia remembers a very wise man telling her that "the year you are born, and the day you pass on are not as important as the dash between the years". So Patricia poses the question "How do you cope with all of life's changes, and not become isolated?"

Coping Without Feeling Isolated

As you age, you must begin to understand that the concept of being "old" is not an instant transition, but a gradual process. When you begin to feel a bit older, you become more reserved and selective of interactions with the people you come into contact with. After some of your friends pass away, you lose part of the ability to articulate how you feel to others, because your mind attempts to remind you that your "time is drawing near".

The most important part is to share your feelings with those around you. Isolation creeps in as you change your behavior, and stop involving people in your life or daily activities.

You should be aware of the need to be included in everything going on around you, and also the need to be in control of it. When you are trying to cope with change, typically you want to control everything in your possession instead of allowing things to happen around you. The best mechanism to deal with change is to embrace and understand it. Break down each item in your life that you feel has evolved and try to place yourself in the present space, rather than the past. Allow others to work with you, primarily family and friends while seeking out others who are going through similar adjustments in life.

When you experience a life-altering event such as death or marriage, it is considered a "rite of passage" (Gennep 1960) (Moody & Sasser 2015). Within certain age ranges you are designed psychologically to take a hard look at your life's decisions and make new strides in, what can be considered, the next journey of your life. The best way to deal with these changes is to understand at an early age that they are inevitable.

Children in the current generation have become more de-sensitized to death and harm, but older adults are more reactive than proactive when it comes to displaying the same agility.

The main objectives are to actively prepare for the next steps, and refrain from isolating yourself. There are people around you that have, or will, experience some of the same revelations in becoming an older adult. Open up, and share the stories and lessons learned.

Isolation is a choice, and choosing not to acknowledge its seriousness is a defense mechanism. Learning how to cope and, in return, alerting others of what to avoid are some of the best and most productive ways to adjust to life's changes.

Key Takeaways:

 Getting old is a gradual process.

 As the body ages, there will be physical changes in the skin, hair, hearing, vision, height and sleep patterns.

 Insomnia may be a sign of depression.

 Recognize changes in behavior and/or feelings of reservation, selective interactions with those you come in contact with on a daily basis, and not wanting to discuss emotions.

 Trying to control everything should be replaced with letting things happen around you.

 Embrace change by not living in the past.

 Find new friends and discuss commonalities.

 Choose not to be alone.

CHAPTER 2

The Conversation

❝ A constant reminder of my age is [me] repeatedly saying, "I'm old. Well, if it's not that extreme, it's the other. I'm over or under dressed, not acting in a civilized manner, and I keep reliving or recreating the memories of the past. I don't want to sit down with you and talk about the next steps in life, I just want to live it!"

This is an excerpt from a conversation I had with an older man after he stormed out of a room away from his children.

Ed was feeling the pressures of everyone present for the discussion, children included, approaching him from all angles. He believed that his loved ones were trying to control his life instead of what was actually happening. His children just wanted him to realize that he wasn't as young as he thought and to be more careful.

Contrary to Ed's reaction is how a woman named Jay handled the intervention style conversation. She was getting ready to sit her children down and explain what she wanted to do after retirement and with the final stages of her life. She had been diagnosed with breast cancer, but was now in remission. Jay recognized that this would be a continuous fight for her life, but her children didn't want to even consider what life would be like without their mother.

Ed and Jay' reactions are what having "the conversation" is all about. What is the best way to approach someone you admire, or look up to and ask that they prepare for, or talk through the *what if's.*

Ed's story is familiar to many. He isn't in a midlife crisis, but wants to do everything he feels he never had a chance to. He wants to recreate all of the moments he missed because he was too busy working at an automobile plant. Time has now caught up with him and he wants to live out his dreams.

Ed's children agree with him, but they want him to live life in a more cautious manner. Ed's family handled this in a way we recommend not doing.

As I spoke with Ed, he described the very moment his children tried to force the notion of him aging down his throat. "It was like yesterday. I walked in the house with vacation tickets for the kids and their families." It had been 4-years since Ed felt the urge to travel, and he believed this was the perfect time. He had beaten the nearly devastating outcomes of a stroke, and knew it was time to explore the world he felt he was missing.

"They asked me to have a seat, similar to the show on TV where you all meet in a room, and everyone pours out their feelings for you, and tells you what they want from you, and you make a choice or they give up on you forever. My son began with: Dad, I get it. You want to visit all the places you were supposed to take mom, but she isn't here. It's healthy for you to have a life, but you have to think about those around you."

Ed sat up and said, "Don't you think I understand that?' I know I need to leave behind some good memories, but I want to have some of my own to remember when you all stick me in a home like we did your mother. She was forgotten and I won't be. Every breath in my body will be lived to fight another day."

His youngest son chimed in, "Dad I call you daily and confirm that you have taken your medications. I manage and attend all appointments along with helping you maintain a healthy diet because we refuse to wait until you are too sick to function. We just want you to recognize that you are 75, not 55. You can't just up and go without a health check or someone knowing how your condition is progressing."

As the conversation concluded, Ed was even more determined to follow his own mind. Ed wanted his kids not to constantly bring up his age, health conditions, or the loss of their mother. His monthly reminder was the bill he paid for her headstone, and the burial plot they both shared. He wanted his life and the remaining days to be similar to his twenties, and he wasn't going to allow any interruptions. What Ed didn't realize is that his children simply wanted him to enjoy life in the safest way possible, and not limit it.

Ed took the vacation with his family and hiked in Europe with some friends. Finally after 3 years of constant movement, he was willing to admit his children were right. Ed said, "I understand what the children meant and the help they offered me. I know back then I was similar to a rebellious teenager, but it was for good reason. I felt as if I had a new chance at life and I took it with no hesitation. My fluid movements were caused by life's regrets and not being able to accept my age and what changes come along with it."

Ed's advice to others is that accepting your age takes time, and you need to accomplish your dreams; otherwise you mentally decline because you are sulking in the notion of *I wish I completed*. Also be mindful that your age does not always determine your lifestyle. Old age is a blessing not a punishment.

In the case with Jay, things played out a bit differently. She sat her children down and wanted to explain how, "Mommy isn't getting any younger, and it is time to take responsibility for you, the family legacy, and me."

Jay's process began with the introduction of insurance paperwork. She was dividing a living trust, preparing a living will, formulating advance care directives, and arranging retirement plans. Her lawyer greeted her four children, while the grandchildren were asked to play in the backyard. Jay's youngest child was 17 years of age and couldn't understand why at 56, his mother was insistent on making plans for the next 10 years.

Kyle argued with his mother, to stop planning her death. She had beaten cancer and life now had a sense of normalcy. The doctor said she was fine and had nothing to worry about, but in her heart, Jay knew her children would not be in the best mental capacity to make any life-lasting decisions. So, she decided to make them for herself.

As she completed all of the work, she began speaking, using her favorite line, "Y'all know I'm getting old now, and it's time to prepare." Her daughter with the same sense of laughter said, "Mom you aren't old. Get over yourself and the nonsense of you dying tomorrow. The doctors all agree you are fine, and the psychologist says that this is just a phase." As her daughter got up to gather her things, Jay demanded in a stern voice, "Sit down and listen!"

Jay told her children that *this conversation* was necessary. She expressed that "although this isn't the best way to have the discussion, we do have guests and they are here to assist us in any way."

After the talk was complete and all documents were signed, Jay told her children, "I am at peace and when the time comes, you need to have this same dialogue amongst yourselves with the children. You all had no idea of what my final wishes were and now you do."

Two years to the day of this faithful speech, Jay passed away. I reached out to her children and they expressed Jay's last sentiment. The children felt that if their mother hadn't shared her plans with them and exactly what she wanted, everything that could have gone wrong would have.

Since they had everything in place, they were able to grieve as a family and prepare seamlessly for the next steps of their lives without their mother. The very last thing they did on their mother's behalf was establishing a legacy fund in honor of end of life planning, for those whose parents want to properly plan, but do not have the means.

So how do you have the conversation with the close family? How do you initiate the conversation with your aging loved ones?

The Chit-Chat

First, you should approach the conversation with love and understanding – knowing your objective, purpose and desired outcome. Anytime you want to speak with someone about aging, ensure that you have a thoughtful process knowing what you want to accomplish. Also, be prepared to share some educational facts about the aging process. Try to account for many perspectives, and not just the idea that you want to present.

Do your research before attempting to intervene with loved ones, and plan to have the discussion during a time where everyone is as open-minded as possible.

You don't want to prolong talking about the next stages in life, or the end of life with your elders, because you may not be able to obtain the answers you are seeking.

For example, if you would like to have an idea of your parent's final wishes, simply ask the question at the right moment. Many elders are in a stage where their loved ones and friends are passing away. Simply say, "I saw the story of your friend, what did or didn't you like about how the family handled their last days?" You may stumble upon the answers you need.

I would also recommend that you take notes, not as they are speaking because you want to be engaged, but after they conclude. Write down their wishes, and maybe in a year or so, try to reconfirm what you have written down. Once the details are confirmed, share with other members of your family so that in the event something happens more than one person has the knowledge of your elder's final arrangements.

Some of the best approaches to gathering information I've seen are questions posed surrounding the elder's opinion, on how friends were treated during the elder stages of life- from beginning to end. If you listen to the comments and stories, you often can distinguish how your loved ones want their final days to play out. After listening, reconfirm and then begin planning your conversation. You have to treat the concept as ongoing and evolving.

Another approach is to inquire how the elder is treating the next stage of life, and what the prospective plans are now that they're retired or no longer doing what they used to do. The end of life is a challenging matter for anyone. When you ask an older person these questions, their first assumption is that you're referring to death. You want to ask the 5 W's; (who, what, when where, why), and express you are looking for a detailed explanation instead of simply answering the basic question, "What are the next steps?" Often times you will find that older adults offer more information when prompted, and as a plus, you present yourself as a listener.

Do not ask, "How do you want to die?" or "who do you want to take over when you are gone?" These questions will immediately result in a shut down and places you further from the answers you need well before you inquire. It isn't ideal to lead a conversation about the ending stages of life just as your loved one leaves the doctor's office, where the notion of aging is ever-so present. Check first to make sure this is not the case, and that their mood isn't potentially darkened by an age-related diagnosis. Gently initiate the discussion, but let them open up to you.

Prior to intervening with the elder, gather the people that are closest to the elder for an initial meeting, and be sure to jot down all key items as everyone shares their viewpoints. You may find that each person has a different piece of valuable information that you will need in order to help the conversation run smoothly.

Some elders may not have close or living relatives that they feel comfortable sharing their final wishes with. As a supportive member of the community or a neighbor, understand that you can serve in that role. Encourage the elder select a family member or offer yourself to be transparent in regards to what they want, and what they believe the next steps should be. If the elder is still hesitant to share final wishes with the family, have the conversation with the elder, being sure to record his or her desires. This way, if something were to happen, you have the necessary details to pass along to family members and friends.

Regardless of relation, every party involved may have different ideals of what's best. When discussing, make sure you understand and value the information shared, and most importantly, respect what the older adult feels. If need be, step away from the conversation if it becomes too combative, but make sure you come back to it when everything has calmed.

Remember, this is an important stage and step in someone's life. Always present the conversation as a session of wisdom and your main objective is to keep the legacy going. No matter the topic – health, safety, final wishes, living arrangements, or finances – give your undivided attention.

Key Takeaways:

 Start the conversation by asking an open-ended question and listen.

 Approach the conversation with dignity; have a purpose and a desired outcome.

 During the conversation, take notes of what is shared and pass along the information to other family members.

 Collaborate with other family members and friends before you initiate the conversation. You may find that you have most of the information you need.

 Take time away from the discussion, and revisit to confirm what you heard.

 Respect the speaker and redirect if the conversation becomes combative.

CHAPTER 3

Someone Else Stepped Up

Kenneth and Dana's Story

Kenneth is a 75- year-old man who has defied the odds with his outrageous habits, and is aging in a successful manner. His story began as he married his second wife. Shortly after this glorious occasion, one of his daughters, along with his wife's daughter, passed away in a fatal accident. Kenneth now suffers from depression, but hides it very well by using laughter, spending time with family, and having a constant sip of alcohol. Kenneth explained that, after a few years his wife began suffering from multiple sclerosis, as she wasn't able to handle the stress of losing his daughter.

Kenneth however, was able to sustain and work at a factory for the next 30 years, until he was forced by the company to retire. Kenneth began having problems with his vision, but was afraid to admit his troubles. In the last 10 years, Kenneth has encountered financial troubles with supporting his remaining children and grandchildren, as well as paying for his wife's medication. The stresses of life, and constantly purchasing new- used vehicles being rundown or totaled by his grandchildren, had interfered with Kenneth's ability to make doctors' appointments and to visit other family members regularly. He noticed his drinking began to increase after the loss of his sister. He made a vow to help those around him, as he was the youngest child and only had one older brother living. Unexpectedly, Kenneth's ex-wife became ill with cancer. Kenneth felt as though their children were not doing enough to help her, so he stepped in to care for her, along with caring for his current wife. Kenneth consistently spent time, effort and money on both households, just as his vision began to deteriorate. Kenneth decided not to give any more time or resources until his children stepped in to help.

As for his own elderly care, Kenneth refused to believe he needed someone to take care of him, and simply stated that he "may be helped, but not taken care of by anyone." Kenneth eventually received that help from an unexpected source. Surprisingly, his granddaughter Dana, who was attending college, decided it was time to step in. She couldn't accurately articulate all of her grandfather's medical conditions, but she helped everyone by creating a schedule for care, spearheading the maintenance medications, and kept everyone, including her step- grandmother, involved actively in the process.

The cycle begins again as Dana steps in to help her family. She sees the need to infuse joy into the lives of those she feels are suffering. She changes universities to be closer to home, and misses out on the ultimate college experience. In her words, "this is a life experience I may need in the future". As Dana completes her last year of school, she has to deal with the death of her step-grandmother and her great-uncle, Kenneth's last and final sibling. Although she is able to move forward, she understands the toll this has taken on her grandparents.

During Dana's last semester of college, Kenneth has injured himself while she was away. Regrettably, Kenneth is now battling with the possibility of losing his eye. Kenneth is cognizant that his drinking has increased, and Dana is concerned that if she doesn't continue to help, her grandfather will assume the responsibility of caring for himself and others again. He may be inclined to ask family members for assistance, ones whom she believes aren't responsible enough to properly care for him.

Dana graduated from school with a bachelor's degree, but is now stuck at a crossroad. She continues to assume the caretaker role that her grandfather relinquished. She is debating accepting a job in a different city, but she doesn't want to bring someone in the home unfamiliar with her family's needs. Will someone else step in?

When you try to fill a void, often times there is another job that will become neglected. Family caregivers have some of the hardest positions, and it is not an elected place to be in. Typically, someone in the family steps up as a caregiver because they are tired or scared of what will come next. In Kenneth's case, and being an older man, he felt it was a necessary to assume full responsibility of taking care of his both his current and ex-wife. Dana, as a younger adult, stepped in because she believed she saw a need. Can you identify when it is your time to step up?

Stepping In & Stepping Up

Due to the many glamorous distractions in today's society, (reality television, plastic surgery, social media, a society that forces elders to deny their age, who try to do everything in their power to be young) many people are unaware that there is a need for aging awareness. Some of the most important factors of this story, and lessons, is the need to be self-aware, attentive to an aging family member's needs, and to be involved with family matters overall. Families disconnecting over small problems or disagreements, or other possible major difficulties, can lead to a lack of participation in caring for the elders. With that said, it is important to be self-aware. Ask yourself the following questions:

 Am I contributing to the issues causing our family to be disconnected?

 Do I play any role in the non-compliance?

 Am I considering the needs of others?

 If you happen to be the elder in need of care: have you evaluated yourself?

 What can I do to open lines of communication, or begin the process of evaluating if there is an actual need?

If I am unable to assist, have I reached out to others, or researched who may be able to help? Especially if the need is medical?

 What are the next steps needed to be taken?

 All of these are viable questions that must be answered in order to step up successfully.

 The next steps are fairly simple:

What is missing?

What can you do to help?

When assisting someone up and down a flight of stairs, or with verbal communication, it is significantly easier to assess and step in; but are you truly watching and understanding everything that is going on around you?

A famous quote reads, "I can't read your mind, but I can read between the lines." And, how this quotation often rings true when it comes to the elder population! Many elders will not come forth to blatantly ask for help, but they will give clues around the subject matter. Calling or stopping by are two of the best ways to help an elder person open up about their needs. Some persons in the older generations have a difficult time adapting to new technology, being alone, transitioning in a different location, and perhaps, receiving help unwarranted. As a younger person it should be a general responsibility to call and ask whether an elder feels safe, and has the basic   necessities such as food, water, shelter and comfort. These particular needs should be met on a continuous basis. The best practice for assessing whether or not there is a basic need is to carefully listen to the elders and observe what is going on around them in their environment, ultimately planning for a way to help. Some needs are obvious and do not warrant analysis.

It is important to share the workload of elder care with other loved ones. If only one person is bearing the majority of the work he or she will inevitably experience what is known as a *"burnout"*. This final lesson is fundamentally rooted in the elder care practice. "Burnout" is a common condition, which can be found in any industry, where one is working, or aiding, for long periods of time without any assistance or breaks.

There are three characterizations to this particular phase. The initial stage is the feeling of guilt or glory. You want to help someone, and it's out of your need to be acknowledged for helping. You become overwhelmed by your task and experience unhappiness; this results in the next stage of finding yourself despising your act of kindness, because you have become exhausted in your efforts and now lack interest.

The next stage in this experience is the feeling of regret. You feel as though there are others around that could help lighten the workload, but they are said to be unavailable. You become spiteful and treat others in rudely, which can all be avoided with a simple conversation to address your feelings.

Care is a team effort, and you have to be able to depend on a group of individuals to assist you. There are always people you can reach out to, and work with helping to care for aging adults. Talk through a plan of rotation so no one experiences a "burnout". Care is an important aspect of an elder's life, and it's essential that all loved ones be mindful of it.

<u>Key Takeaways:</u>

 A family caregiver is a responsible person who is willing to adjust his or her own schedule to help.

 A family caregiver should involve other loved ones in creating an active plan of care for the elder.

 Be aware of the elder's needs by calling and making well-check visits.

 Put aside family disagreements to help your elders.

 If you are not the main caregiver, make it your mission to assist with elder care to help lessen the chances of a "burnout". Volunteering to transport or doing some house cleaning are just a couple of examples of how you can help.

 Caregiving involves being a companion.

 Being a caregiver is a loving and passionate act.

CHAPTER 4

The Sandwich Generation

The *sandwich generation* is a phrase that was created in order to illustrate when an adult is wedged between caring for elderly parents and young children. Dorothy Miller, creator of the ideal, also breaks down the sandwich generation into subsets: *the sandwich, open sandwich* or *the club sandwich*. The sandwich generation is defined as being in your thirties and forties caring for young children and your older parents. The *"open"* sandwich generation is similar except it is any loved one, not just limited to parents. The club sandwich generation describes elder adults caring and providing a level of stability for their children and grandchildren. Unbeknownst to Beverly, military mom of a 12-year-old and two 5-year-olds, she fell into the open sandwich subset.

Aside from being a busy mother, Beverly also owns and operates a video and photography studio. She primarily assisted with wedding parties, but recently a selection of her photographs caught the eye of a famous collector. Because of the growth in her career, she began to travel every other month for more photography jobs. Her husband, Randall, has been enlisted in the armed services for over 25 years, and currently has active orders. Beverly's immediate family moved approximately every two years, but this particular move was a bit different. Her mother-in-law had fallen ill and Beverly's dad was diagnosed with cancer. Initially, Beverly had the unique conversation on what should be done; first with herself, then with health care providers, and finally with her husband. Upon meeting with a company of eldercare consultants, she was given an advance care plan, legal, and financial advice for her parents.

Beverly's story is not uncommon, but is definitely an extreme case. After the passing of her mother almost 10 years ago, Beverly realized that she didn't get to see her father as often as she liked. Subsequently, her father adjusted to life fairly well but was stuck in his ways, and was set on not leaving Seattle. He was involved in his church organizations, played golf with his senior friends and came to see the kids when he took time off from his post retirement job at a fishing port. He longed to be closer to some of his family members in Georgia, but they would often come and visit him.

When Beverly learned of her father's diagnosis, she felt as though this would be the perfect opportunity to have him come and live close by; he could help keep order around the house and with the kids. She lived in a large home in northern California and knew this would be her husband's last tour. She was convinced that having her father move in was a great idea and she presented it to the family. Her husband agreed, and after a few weeks her dad agreed as well.

Beverly's father moved into the guesthouse after his last round of treatments, and his recovery was progressively positive. Beverly was in a good place, knowing that all the details were working out.

Six months later, Randall came to the family with news that his own mother was experiencing heart complications and showing signs of dementia. Martha was 88 and said that she wanted to see her grandchildren more often. Randall wasn't too sure if having his mother move in was an option, seeing as he already agreed to have Beverly's father live in the guesthouse. Supportively, Beverly insisted that she could take a back seat in her profession and her father would be there to lend an extra set of helping hands in the care of Randall's mother.

Not all families have a plan such as this work in their favor, but both Beverly and Randall seemed to manage just fine, even with opinionated parents around.

About a year into the arrangement, Beverly began feeling overwhelmed. She said that taking care of both parents' needs was becoming increasingly difficult, while also managing a teenager and small children. Balancing doctor's appointments, special diet requests, children's schedules, and her business, began to take a toll on her. She was taking care of six people, apparently on her own, and didn't know what her next steps should be.

Beverly researched several gated, senior living facilities and nursing homes in her neighborhood for her father and mother-in-law. She felt as if this may have been the right time to move the parents into a place where there was care readily available, so she could spend more time balancing her life. Her dad stopped driving due to his vision deteriorating, and became increasingly confrontational with her and the children. Randall's mom became more and more forgetful, along with having limited mobility. Beverly sat her husband down and explained that the last four years of her life had been a blur of restrictions, because both the children and parents needed her undivided attention. She felt caught in the middle most days, trying to do what was best for her children, and accepting the harsh criticism from her parents and family, because she wasn't able to manage the constant needs of her family, and the demands of her career.

Beverly laid out a plan that she believed everyone in the family would agree with. She included her father's youngest sister and her mother-in-law's ex-husband. They all lived within a 20-mile radius, and Beverly felt it was a win for the entire group. She succeeded, and so her parents lived another 4 years without incident.

Her father moved into a gated community where his sister decided to live as well. Meanwhile, Beverly's ex-father-in-law pulled some strings to get his ex-wife into a home where he could visit daily.

Eventually, Beverly's husband retired from the military and was able to stay home with the kids, giving Beverly an opportunity to get back to doing what she loved.

Beverly explained that, from the inside, it seemed like the days were long; multiple opportunities were overlooked, and she felt like she missed some major moments in her kid's lives. Beverly's oldest daughter, Ashley, shared how she saw her mother doing something no other person would dream of. She professed how proud she was of her mother.

Beverly explained that she wasn't the only one she knew of who took care of their parents, while still raising small children. In fact, she went on to encourage others to do the same. She described the importance of performing such an act of selflessness while loved ones are healthy.

Beverly's story is an example of the best-case scenario. If you happen to find yourself in a similar situation, make sure to have an exit strategy, and consider all possible outcomes when in the planning stages. Not everyone is willing to take someone into his or her home, and care for multiple family members in need. For those already caring for small children, some of the most common concerns prior to taking on the care of elders are:

How do I survive living in this sandwich generation?

Are others having this issue? If so, what is their plan?

Surviving the Sandwich generation

Dorothy Miller was a pioneer in the aging generation; she is the primary reason why the current society understands what the sandwich generation is. When trying to navigate your way through the process, there are a few items that you should think about before, during, and after you are tasked with caring for a loved one. One of the first things you need to do is create a plan. Assessing your financial state is a key component. Look at funding from your retirement funds, investments and family expenses.

401K and Roth funds are amazing ways to save money, but what are some other means? Can you invest in an insurance policy or in the stock market, so that you can make additional funds outside of what you are saving right now? Be mindful that modern medicine and healthy living have extended life expectancy, so plan for that and reserve your assets.

Being a part of the sandwich generation can be an extraordinary experience for the parental caregivers. They will get to witness, firsthand, the wisdom instilled in them as children, being taught directly from their parents to their own children: valuable lessons that are often times lost within a family's history.

Key Takeaways:

 The Sandwich Generation refers to those who care for elderly loved ones and their own young children, simultaneously.

 Now is the time to create a plan of care for yourself and your family through crucial conversations.

 Be sure to spend as much time as possible with the children.

 Create a back-up plan for your finances.

Save now using Roth or 401K funds. Invest in stocks and insurance policies.

 With advance care planning, it's important to be proactive, and not reactive.

 Always consult professionals when developing financial or healthcare plans

CHAPTER 5

Drugs for what? By whom?

"Hand me the small white pill, and the big gray pill!" she exclaimed. "Well, no! Wait! I took that, but my back hurts. Hand me those Aleve." I sat and observed a woman named Louise referencing her pills by color. I wanted to know who was helping her, or monitoring the drugs she was consuming. I first met Louise at a local pharmacy counter where she handed me a pill container from 1988. It was for her husband and she wanted to get the prescription renewed. She meekly explained that her husband had just run out of his blood pressure medication. I asked Louise if it was all right for me to assist her and she exclaimed, "Yes! I've been needing some help with these drugs." Louise was 92 years old and her husband, John, was 93. She explained how they were an ideal team. She out lived their only daughter, and had no grandchildren. She used the local bus service to get around, and lived in a gated community where the neighbors primarily helped her and her husband around the apartment. I had so many questions for Louise, but I took the time to sit with her as she shared her story, dating back 15 years.

Louise and her husband are in decent health, but over the last 5 months, Louise's health has been on a decline. She could remember most things, but the regimen of her medications was getting the best of her. Louise and her husband walked every day around the community from 11 a.m. until about 12:30 p.m., which they considered to be their daily exercise; and ate three to four meals a day, never missing the ice cream shop on the corner for a shared scoop of mint chocolate chip.

Movement was often slow, and to subside, Louise depended on her pills aligned on the kitchen counter, paired with a color-coded directory matching the pills to her ailments. After her husbands' retirement from Lincoln Electric, the pair moved from their large home in Ohio and took up residence in Texas, where Louise was a homemaker who tailored clothes for prominent executives' downtown. They both decided, since Dallas was where they met, that it would be the perfect place for them to grow old together.

Louise walked into a pharmacy in 1988 with a prescription for her husband to treat high blood pressure. At the time, the medication was new on the market and they couldn't afford it with their Medicaid. She asked for a 3-month supply of the medication, because she knew it would last.

She was given 100 pills and decided to cut them into fifths because her husband refused to take any medication. After days of forgetting to have her husband take medication, or simply not breaking the pills because she couldn't find the pill splitter, Louise ended up with over twenty years' worth of expired medication. Now, any medical professional will tell you the hazards of taking expired medication. Frankly, you aren't supposed to take medication after it expires, but unfortunately for Louise, no date was listed on the bottle. In turn, she just kept up with her normal routine – a few home remedies and maybe a pill or two– and insisted that she was able to care for herself and her husband until she became ill.

Louise, had been diagnosed with heart failure, which came with a number of complications. She was hospitalized in the late 2000's and was told to take a plethora of medications in order to survive. After deliberating with her husband, Louise agreed to follow the doctor's orders, and began going to the local pharmacy every Tuesday afternoon at 2 p.m. to pick up her prescriptions, and one day she finally remembers her husband's pills just ran out.

She was a favorite customer of all the locals, and no one ever questioned how she kept up with life. Three specialists saw Louise frequently for her heart, and she kept a number of regular appointments with a few other doctors. Managing between doctors became difficult, so every week she took a piece of paper and wrote down each doctor's name with a color next to it, identifying which pill she should take and who prescribed it to her. The next column outlined how many times she should take the medication. One of the most difficult parts of the day for Louise was remembering the proper dosage to take for her blood thinner. Every other week the dosage would change due to the results of her blood test, known as INR. Due to the nature of her condition, she knew she could not cure herself with "tussin" or Alka-Seltzer, as she once could before.

Over the coming months, the pharmacy changed distributors, and it has become increasingly difficult to find the medication with the similar colors that she was used to. I asked Louise what would happen if she lost her color-coded tracker. She explained how she'd lost it a few times before, and if she were unable to find it; she would simply follow the directions from the previous week, and would write down new instructions for the weeks to come.

The moment of frustration came when she visited the pharmacy only to find that her medication changed, yet again. She wanted to search for another doctor and pharmacist, and coincidently, her husband reminded her that he hadn't been to the doctor recently, and was also in need of getting his prescription filled.

Louise brought her husband's old prescription bottle to the pharmacy counter and said, "I think his doctor is still alive, but you should check." Louise's main concern was how could she keep the details of their doctors, pharmacies, and medications straight?

Keeping the Medications in Order

According to the medical dictionary, Polypharmacy is a term that refers to the effects of taking multiple medications concurrently to manage co-existing health conditions. Typically, heart patients are the most common to experience this issue. When you have multiple doctors and there isn't an interdisciplinary care plan, medications, along with conditions, become subdued. Medications are over prescribed, and patients lose track of which of their conditions needs to be constantly monitored. Ways to help tackle this problem begin with you and continue with your physician.

In a typical practice, your primary care doctor will refer you to a specialist specifically for your medical condition. Once you have met with the specialist, and depending on the health risks, there are follow-ups with other physicians as well as circling back with previous doctors. Directed in all discharge paperwork from hospitals or clinics is to schedule a follow-up appointment with your primary care physician, a step that is neglected by some patients far too often.

The best way to counter this problem is for the patient to develop a team care plan. This resource houses all points of contact needed for the patient and each member involved in the particular stage of care. To start, the best approach is to list each physician you visit currently, including the reasons for the doctor's visits, and diagnosis. The next step for developing a team care plan is to add the pharmacy or any herbalist that you may contact concerning your health. Directly after this step, you should allow the doctors to add notes that they may have from any procedures, or notes referencing any health issues.

You will then need to provide a direct contact to a pharmacy of your choice. All of this information should be found in your electronic medical record, and shared with those closest to you in a paper form.

The final step in developing a team care plan is to review the plan with loved ones contributing to care. You will often find that medications have been duplicated, unnecessary procedures were administered, no follow-up appointment was ever created with the primary care physician, and there is a limited record of the patient summary visit from other facilities.

Having a second line of communication open with a family member, or friend, that understands your health needs is essential to this plan being efficient. They would have access to your medical information, and would be able to report back to the physician and pharmacists on your status, if ever needed.

Key Takeaways:

 Polypharmacy occurs when medications are taken concurrently to manage a health condition.

 Seeing numerous physicians can potentially lead to multiple prescriptions that may not be monitored properly.

 Always follow-up with your primary doctor after you have visited any specialist or new physician. Be sure to read and follow the instructions outlined in your discharge paperwork when released from doctor's care.

 Your care team includes doctors, pharmacists, herbalists. You should notify each group of any significant changes.

 Create a simplified interdisciplinary care plan for yourself, and review it with your care team.

 Have a second line of communication with a family member or close friend, who can articulate your needs and has access to the simplified care plan.

CHAPTER 6

My House: Can I Stay?

Melba is a unique woman who exerts every ounce of compassion and kindness to others, but lives in fear of being outside. Melba's story is common and creates an avenue for examining housing situations of our elders. Melba currently lives in a long-term care facility that isn't up to her standards, but her insurance covers the cost. It is located in a neighborhood that is close to where she grew up, and accommodates the living arrangements for herself, her mother, and her daughter. Melba's story begins with her 8th grade education, and the fact that the daycare facility where she worked suggested she retire due to constant absences for caregiving reasons. Melba was the sole provider for her two children, two grandchildren, a living mother, and a husband, now deceased. She lived in the inner city close to where she grew up as a child. She is 85-years-old, and now her son, and granddaughter, are her only living family members.

Melba shows signs and symptoms of a declining mental acuity after the traumatic experience of transitioning to a long-term care facility. She was able to tell her story with the help of her caregiver adding in details that Melba has blocked from memory, as a result of her emotional attachment. Melba's story began after she retired from the daycare and was able to receive social security, along with retirement from her job and her husband's pension. Two years prior to retirement, Melba's daughter was diagnosed with multiple sclerosis and moved in with her. Melba did not want any outside caregivers in the home, so she took on the responsibility of caring for her daughter on her own. Initially, caring for her daughter took up much of Melba's time, because she had to make the necessary adjustments to her home in order to transition it into a handicap accessible space. Melba took classes and studied books on her daughter's condition to better educate herself. During this process and within the very next year, Melba's mother fell ill, and so she made the decision to take her in as well. This living arrangement was the most cost effective, and reduced the stress of constantly checking on ill family members who lived in two different places. As Melba approached retirement and her home became dilapidated, she realized that her living arrangement was no longer in the best of conditions to safely care for her handicapped loved ones.

Melba's retirement proved to be helpful as she was able to stay home to care for her mother and daughter on a daily basis; but she was unaware of the rapid decline of the home's aesthetic, both interior and exterior, and cleaning was unfortunately not a top a priority. She began receiving complaints about the compost in the back yard and the neglectful lawn care. After a visit from the city workers, Melba was convinced that she could take care of the needs herself. Over the next 6 months, her daughter became severely ill and passed away in the home. Melba became depressed and barely had the strength to complete the tasks that her mother asked of her. The home became severely disheveled and the housing authority, office of the aging, and pet authorities were all contacted. Forced to move out of the home because the city and state deemed it unlivable, Melba and her mother now depended on the assistance from their assigned caseworker for a new housing placement. These series of events left Melba traumatized because she no longer had control over her estate, which was once paid in full. Armed with only an 8th grade education, Melba wasn't privy to the required measures the city and state had to take in order to move residents out of their homes.

At 63 years of age, Melba, with her mother, moved into a long-term care facility that was close to her childhood neighborhood; and for the next 15 years, they shared a living space in a subsided area of an eight-bedroom facility, until Melba's mother attempted to harm her. The pair was separated into single bedrooms, but continued to share common living areas for another two years. It was at that moment, Melba realized that she hadn't been away from her mother in years. Melba's initial feelings were of freedom and relaxation because she could be totally released from care, but after several months that excitement turned to sadness. Melba's purpose was to care for her mother and this had been taken away.

Her son would come to visit, but had resentment because he was unable to gain ownership of their family home from the state. He was a reformed drug user and knew that his mother's and grandmother's current living conditions were not much better than the previous arrangement, but it was all the family could afford. Melba's mom passed away after living in the facility for 17 years, leaving Melba as one of four residents currently in the space.

On occasion, Melba would venture outside of the home for outings and appointments, but an accident - a slip and fall - stopped her from leaving the property. Her normal routine now consists of standing in the doorway to receive fresh air once or twice every four months, and walking around inside with a small radio for entertainment. She stands in the doorway for the occasional season change, but will not step 2 feet away from the door.

I asked Melba to describe her experience. Simply stated, she says that over the last 22 years of her life, she has seen people come and go. With my experience, I understood the family's housing situation. However, Melba never fully grasped how it happened. The question she consistently asks everyone she's interacted with is: how can anyone take your home, or remove you if you feel that it is in your best interest to stay?

Time to Relocate

The housing authority is a pretentious organization that establishes the guidelines of where your home is located, and how the property and land is managed; unfortunately, they have the capacity to remove anyone who is non-compliant with the guidelines. Each state gives a different level of control to housing authorities; however, the federal government is able to step in and claim eminent domain in the event your space needs to be occupied. As citizens, it is important that everyone is aware of the housing laws in your municipality and knows where the local office is situated.

There are many misconceptions in regards to the process in which your home can be taken away from you. It begins with complaints, which are then turned into a written petition. The occupants are summoned to appear in court and given a chance to fix their home, making sure that it is compliant with the housing authority's guidelines. If the occupants choose not to adhere to the judge's ruling, the option to stay will be taken.

Next, is the appealing process: according to court documents, appeals can take years to process, and residents typically give in to the housing authority's demands.

The best advice from Melba when dealing with this situation is to be mindful of your living conditions, and understand that standards and conduct are subject to the opinion of others. Even if the home is yours it is subject to codes and regulations surrounding one's care. It will be taken away by the city if it doesn't follow city-defined ordinances.

If you could no longer live at home, where would you go? Who would you call?

Initially, one should contact their local Agency on Aging or the Division of Senior and Adult Services. Here, you will be able to get a geriatric social worker to assess your needs. The agency can help make recommendations of the best possible and safe environment for you to live.

Key Takeaways:

 Call ADULT PROTECTIVE SERVICES, if needed.

 Call the police if there is a safety issue with an elderly person or the community involved.

 Look for alternative housing through local agencies.

 ADULT FAMILY CARE (AFC) homes are offered to individuals who are no longer able to live alone. They have the opportunity to move in and share the home with a caretaker who is capable of providing needed assistance and supervision.

 ACCESSORY APARTMENTS are units, which have been added onto or created within a single-family house. It allows older persons to live independently, but close to people who care for them.

 ADULT RETIREMENT COMMUNITIES are specifically designed for active, independent elders. Units are generally for purchase, but occasionally rental units are available.

 ASSISTED LIVING RESIDENCES - (ALR) - are licensed by the Department of Health. This care is intended to promote maximum independence for residents with 24-hour assistance.

CONTINUING-CARE RETIREMENT COMMUNITIES - (CCRC) - provide housing, services, healthcare, and nursing home care to elders.

 HOME SHARING is a living arrangement in which two or more unrelated people share the common areas of a house.

 NURSING HOMES are residential facilities that provide 24-hour supervision by licensed nurses.

 RESIDENTIAL HEALTH CARE FACILITIES - (RHCF) - are facilities that provide health maintenance and monitoring services under the direction of a professional nurse.

HOW SAFE IS YOUR LOVED ONE

Below is a list of questions that you can refer to when assessing the safety level of your loved one's residence. If you discover that your loved one is in immediate danger call 911, and/or Adult Protective Services to have a full assessment completed, and to determine the appropriate following steps for the elder.

1. Is the environment they reside in clean and healthy?

2. Can they dial 911 or recognize danger?

3. Will they wander away from home and return safely?

4. Will they be able to exit the home or are they bound by a multitude of confusing locks on the doors and windows?

5. Do they understand how to leave the home if necessary? Do they know where the door is located and how to exit the building?

6. Can they re-enter the home with ease by locating the door?

7. Are they self-medicating correctly?

8. Are they able to feed or toilet themselves?

9. Will they let in strangers?

10. Are safe activities planned for them daily?

CHAPTER 7

Guardianship: Who is in Control?

C ontrol is an ambiguous term that can be manipulated by government entities, in the event you are unable to speak for yourself. Guardianship is a topic often missed in the advance care planning conversation, because it usu- ally surfaces as a last resort. Monetary restrictions are regularly the determining factor of who gains guardianship, and more than often the result is the family leaves on adverse terms.

Mark is currently residing in an assisted living facility and although he is battling dementia, he is able to share his story, which is as vivid as if it were today. I sat next to Mark in a courthouse, and couldn't help but notice that he seemed to be emotionally disturbed. At the beginning of our interaction, his opening line caught me by surprise. "I always thought I had control over my life, but maybe not." Out of anger, he burst into tears exclaiming, "I want the best for me, and if it has to be by force, so be it!"

Mark has two sons and one daughter. Mark's wife passed away several years prior to this event, as a result of complica- tions from a stroke. Mark is a diabetic and recently had a foot amputation. He was able to get around the house fairly well, and continued working with the caretaker from home health agency that assisted his wife. Sheryl primarily helped Mark with his wife prior to her passing, and afterwards decided to stay to help Mark through his process of healing. Sheryl was great around the family and his daughter was very appreciative of her. The concern surfaced when Mark decided to amend his will because his wife was no longer alive. He had been an executive of a large company and was fairly wealthy.

Mark felt that because Sheryl had done so much with the family, she was now a part of it and deserved a monetary gift for her service. Mark's sons did not express the same sentiments. Mark had approximately $3,000,000 in life insurance and about $10,000,000 in wealth and assets. Mark's sons were not as well-off, working dead end jobs, and according to Mark, they knew a large portion of Mark's estate would be left to them in the event he wasn't able to speak for himself, or passed away. Mark's sons feared there would be a decrease in their financial inheritance, if another person grew close to their father. Once their mother passed, Mark amended the will to include her portion of insurance funds received. Although Mark didn't express his sentiments about adding Sheryl to his life insurance policy with his family, his next few encounters with his sons would prove to him that everyone didn't have his best interest at heart. So Mark updated his will but didn't change his power of attorney.

In the late fall of 2013, Mark presented Sheryl with a check and defended her recent inclusion into the living will. This angered his sons, and so they decided to freeze all of his assets, marking the beginning of a long and unpleasant fight over money. One of his sons hired a lawyer, and since his name was secondary on all the bank accounts, he was able to temporarily freeze the assets. This all began after Mark had notified them that he had updated his living will.

Mark's sons felt that Sheryl was manipulating him into giving her money and so her contracted was terminated. Lisa, Mark's daughter, lived in Paris with her small, but growing family. She had a stepdaughter named Ann, who lived in the house with Mark while continuing her education in California. Ann was similar to a child living in the home. She knew how to care for Mark and sometimes stepped in when asked, however, she was an older college student. She contributed to the household and treated Mark like her grandfather but essentially her biggest role didn't come until the court appearance. After long court battles, coupled with mandatory psychological examinations, the judge understood that no one person seemed to have Mark's best interest at heart except Ann. The judge awarded his step-granddaughter with guardianship. The judge determined that Ann seemed to be the only one focused on Mark's declining health and his best wishes.

Prior to this decision, Ann brought her grandfather to school to participate in an advanced care plan for a collegiate project. She got him to document all of his desired wishes and needs, in the event no one would listen to him or would fight over his wealth. During the hearing, Ann presented this document to the judge and explained that since her grandfather gave her an opportunity to finish school and begin a career without accumulating too much debt, she wanted to return the favor. Ann felt as if no one was paying attention to his lapses in thought or judgment, or to the fact that his care and health rapidly declined as the argument over his money ensued.

Ann's role as his guardian was to find him a safe environment to live, and make sure he continued to see his doctor on a regular basis. Mark understood what was going on around him, and wasn't resistant to the fact that someone be appointed to speak on his behalf and make decisions for him; he just never imagined that his voice wouldn't act as the final say in those decisions.

Thanks to Ann's help, Mark was able to understand that a five-bedroom home with multiple levels wasn't the safest place for him to be, and living alone was not in his best interest. Together Mark and Ann found adequate housing. Mark stopped driving due to a decline in vision but quickly adjusted. He expressed that not having driving privileges wasn't a punishment, but more of a freedom. Services and goods could be delivered to him according to his needs, and creating a weekly to-do list helped with formulating his day. Mark used his sense of business and planning to help manage his own personal life. The guardian protected Mark from his family members with ill intentions, and from them potentially using his money and influence in the community against him.

Mark's pieces of advice and questions were simple: Can you avoid having a guardian? If not, how can you be sure that the courts appoint the person with the best intentions for your life?

If you have someone who is now speaking and deciding on your behalf, do you still have control over your life?

Staying in Command

Guardianship is typically a last resort, and comes into play when families cannot agree on the best resolution for an elder who may be suffering from any stages of Alzheimer's and dementia. In some cases, these particular elders have been deemed unfit to make adequate decisions for themselves, and the family cannot determine who has the best interest of their loved one. Making the decision of who should be in control is never easy, especially when the elder is opposing a close member of the family.

When you have to allow the courts to make the best decision for you, the feeling of loss of control is eminent, and the elder may shut down or become unwilling to move forward. One of the first things you should do with older adults in a scenario where they believe their choices are being challenged is to suggest certain decision outcomes with the right approach. It is imperative to consider day-to-day activities and safer methods that will benefit their day. Driving is one of the hardest habits to give up. Elders are more inclined to relinquish driving privileges when presented with other means of transportation, than having the freedom forcibly revoked. Encourage older adults to use transportation services or delivery services, instead of having to maintain their personal vehicle. It's a way to prompt better driving habits while maintaining independence. As the caregiver, don't take over the driving unless you have the capacity to do so. Share with your elder the new means of technology that can make running errands a little easier. For example: placing an order for delivery via phone or mobile apps, exploring in-home doctors' visits options, or considering hiring an elder driving service. These methods can subtly transition the daily responsibilities to a different party, without giving up the sense of freedom to roam about the city.

The next step is to find a neutral person willing to handle your affairs. When you have a guardianship hearing the state or county chooses and agent to be the decision maker, the older adult essentially is now considered a minor. Since Mark experienced his family challenging his decisions, there was no choice but to assign someone to make decisions on Mark's behalf. In Mark's case he already had someone in mind that, if given the choice for someone to speak on his behalf, it would be someone he was familiar with and neutral to the parties fighting. If there is a challenge in the order of your affairs, try using an agent that has been selected by the older adult who is neutral. It will be a simpler process to gain buy-in, than being assigned someone with no familiarity of the case or family. Being aware of the laws in your city and state is always helpful, and finding a means to collect information surrounding how the process works can be obtained from adult service centers, adult daycares and office of the aging.

Guardianship is a far-reaching step to take. Like Mark's experience, it may become a long process with several proceedings through the courts. It is important to understand that there are various types of guardians, and the differences between them all. Some that are commonly used are *guardian of a person*, where they make decisions for personal and healthcare; and *a guardian of the estate*, who will make financial and legal decisions. *Plenary*, better known as full guardianship, executes all decisions as ordered by the courts. *Limited guardianship* will allow the elder to maintain some say and perform some duties, while the *assigned court guardian* may only perform duties outlined by the court. A *temporary guardianship* will be used for emergencies where there is an immediate danger or threat to the elder.

You may ask, "What happens if the appointed guardian cannot perform the duties assigned?" There is hope! A *standby guardian* may step up to the position, but will need to petition the court to become the *successor guardian*. Many states view a guardian as the person who handles personal affairs, as opposed to a conservator who manages financial and estate affairs. In some cases, there may be a need to assign more than one guardian, who will then become *co-guardians*. Whatever the case, an assigned guardian must follow the law or they can be removed.

<u>Key Takeaways:</u>

 Create a care plan that can be followed by a Guardian, in the event someone is appointed.

 Make decisions early on in the process of aging so the older adult feels as if their wishes are being heard.

 When decision making, propose a plethora of options and opportunities so the elder doesn't feel as if they are being controlled.

 In the event you suspect financial exploitation, review and document all instances while recording behavior that does not fall within their typical spending pattern.

 Speak with attorneys who specialize in older adults and estate affairs for guidance.

CHAPTER 8

My Mind is Sharp

How many times are you going to ask me "am I all right?" Ester shouted. Her daughter Sydney explained that her mother's random outbursts were becoming more frequent, but were controllable. As Ester turned to me, she asked for the fifth time, "What is your name and what do you want to talk about, girl? I have to go to the store and I need to stand by the door for my husband Arthur." I smiled and said, "I want to hear about some of your greatest accomplishments." She smiled back and told me that it would be a long afternoon but that she had time.

Ester has been battling early stages of Alzheimer's ever since she turned 72 years old. The first signs were small. She would forget where she placed her keys, or ask about clothing three or four times such as where her daughter purchased a pair of shoes or a handbag from. Ester's condition progressively worsened as years passed. Sydney was not familiar with the disease, its progression, or what onset symptoms looked like. So, she sometimes had difficulty accepting that her mother seemed to greet her as a new person every few days. Sydney has going through personal counseling to overcome the guilt of her mother's digressing state. She always believed that if she had encouraged her mother to see a physician sooner, or had her mother practice puzzles that could have helped with her memory, she could have prevented the rapid decline.

In order to help bring awareness to the effects of aging, Sydney now advocates for children and loved ones in the neighborhood to pay attention to the signs and symptoms of Alzheimer's, and encourages family members to ask their parents prompting questions about health.

Ester is now 72-years-old, and keeps up with the same daily routine. She awakens at 5:45 a.m., walks the circular path of the long-term care facility, sits and enjoys breakfast with Mrs. Nancy, a resident in the facility, and finally waits at the front door for her husband to visit. Every Sunday, Sydney lays out her mom's clothing for the upcoming week, labeling the outfits by days; brings new books to read, and medications for the nurses to give. She explains how keeping routines helps to combat the memory loss. She wants her mother to have a great quality of life even though her condition will inevitably worsen.

Sydney is very involved in her mother's care and visits the facility unannounced during the week. She feels that this is the best way to determine if staff's daily responsibilities, in regards to her mother's care, are being performed. Due to her mother skepticism of a need for an immediate knee replacement surgery, she walks slower and it is hard for her to move up and down stairs. "Mom loves the path, because it helps her cope with the transition of moving out of her home", says Sydney.

As Arthur approaches, he hugs his wife and tells her, "Let's go for a walk again to fall in love like we used to." Once they leave, Sydney explains that after teaching for the local university for over 35 years, one day her mother forgot an assignment for class and dismissed the students. For the remainder of the semester she would have more moments such as this one, forgetting to tell students important information and asking about it in the next session. It was her last year of teaching, and Ester retired not knowing that she was in the premature stages of Alzheimer disease.

Over the next couple of months, moments like this became even more frequent, until her husband asked Sydney if she ever thought that her mom was beginning to get sick. As Sydney tears up she says, "I remember going to the doctors with her for a series of tests. Days later we were seeing a neurologist. As we were given directions on what the next steps were, my mother simply said, 'I know your father, and he won't be able to care for me as I need, so we need to make the plans now to be successful.'" The following weeks were a series of whirlwinds to find an assisted living facility with memory care available, as well as planning for the end of life. Sydney formulated a plan and was thankful for the counseling available to help strategize the next steps for her family.

Sydney helped her parents move into an assisted living facility not far from their home. She appreciated how easy the process was: her mother had always been open to receiving help from others.

Her parents share an apartment and her mother is constantly monitored by the facility. When it becomes too difficult to monitor his wife or care for her in their small residence, Ester can move to a different section of the building for memory care. She currently visits all of the adults residing on that floor, and is still able to read. She forgets words, phrases, and some basic functions, but overall, she is living a moderately normal life; and has reminders set on her Apple Watch to eat, walk, and read, in order to help make her day run even smoother.

Ester shared the story of her early years, and how instead of pursuing her dream of becoming a ballerina, she was prompted by her family to become a teacher. After becoming an English professor, Ester won several awards writing short stories. She says one of her favorite memories was reading to Sydney, and watching her begin to read in return. She says that some days she can remember everything, but others are a struggle. Ester wants to do what's best for her family, and believes that they love her. She accepts that her memory is fading and opens up about what she wants next. Ester frequently apologizes for repeating herself, and then moves about her day normally.

Sydney shared her story to many older adults, and families in the facility, the devastating effects of Alzheimer's and its unraveling effect it can have on the family. Sydney worries about her father's conditions and his emotions as he himself, witnesses his wife change drastically. Her father attends weekly therapy sessions, and reads articles from the doctor's office about what he can do to hold on to whom he grew to know as his wife. Sydney is aware that other families deal with similar challenges and has found ways to be supportive. Sydney donates to the Dementia and Alzheimer's Research that looks for cures and participates in events that bring awareness. Sydney also participates in family and friend support groups. She sometimes is disturbed by their shared stories and regrets not stepping in or talking to her mother's physicians about the changes prior to her condition becoming what it is now. Sydney often asks herself "What could I have done during the initial moments when I noticed mom's behavior was changing?"

Monitor the Mind

Alzheimer's and dementia are two of the most commonly identified brain disorders within the elderly community. The signs and symptoms are noticeable, however the acceptance of these conditions is difficult for sufferers and their families. There are medications that can be taken to help delay some of the symptoms, but no cure for either one of the diseases.

One of the most important steps in the process of aging, more specifically when dealing with a memory loss disease, is a proper diagnosis and treatment plan that can be executed immediately. Some older adults are misdiagnosed with dementia or Alzheimer's because of their outward behavior towards others in society. In order to be diagnosed, multiple blood tests and brain scans must be conducted however financial limitations or insurance constraints, can cause this step to sometimes be skipped. When this happens, it becomes a misrepresentation of the disease and older adults can be misdiagnosed. Older adults may not always have a memory loss disease, but simply a loss of zeal when it comes to performing the daily activities in life.

According to the Alzheimer's Association, there are many different types of dementia, including vascular, mixed, Parkinson's disease dementia, and Huntington's disease; and there are also early warning signs to look for when monitoring older adults. Skill performance with (ADLs) activities of daily living is an in-home assessment that can be observed. Look for symptoms, such as difficulty remembering times or places, visual images, and relationships, day-to-day tasks within the work place or asking multiple questions on the same subject repetitively. There can be difficulty with speech or recalling facts, having trouble identifying the correct verbiage when discussing topics, misplacing items, or not being able to follow a pattern of behavior – just to name a few.

If you notice that your elder is showing a few of the signs listed, the best approach is to initiate the conversation. As referenced in chapter two, approaching the intervention with the notion of sustaining the elder's legacy is a surefire way to get them to open up about the end of life. Don't forget: bringing up the passing of a relative or neighbor may help to spark the conversation as well.

After making doctor's appointments to get a confirmed and corrected diagnosis, hiring an eldercare consultant to complete the advance care plan should follow. Then, you or a family member along with a professional need to assess whether the home of the elder is a safe environment. If you need to hire additional support, or schedule follow-ups with a home health aide, determine how many resources are in your area. Be sure to interview the potential individuals who will work in your home.

If the home is deemed unsafe, choose a facility that accommodates memory care, and see if your insurance will be able to cover some of the moving expenses into the facility of choice. Remember to keep all family members involved in decision-making, and create a schedule to monitor all appointments, daily needs, and important deadlines. Creating a living will and advance directives for family to follow prior to the decline of all cognitive functions is crucial.

There are many preventative measures that can be taken in order to delay the onset of any of the deteriorating symptoms. Creating puzzles, reading or studying, and activities with smaller children are some of the most profound interventions that are successful. Planning and formulating a care plan are crucial and vital steps when assisting in the process. Ignoring habits, or behavior, will only serve to accelerate the progression of the disease because you are not taking medication or participating in activities to slow the progression. Visit a specialist or physician that practices with elder patients. It is the best choice, and insurance plans may offer therapy for coping with the disease, which is also important for overall health and acceptance.

Sydney now has more than enough information to help others who exhibit the same concerns within her family. She is prepped and willing to assist relatives with prevention strategies.

Key Takeaways:

 Create a plan before a crisis arises. Gracefully involve the family in discussing an advanced care plan.

 As an elder, be proactive and create activities that exercise the mind and memory.

 Look for difficulty in performing activities of daily living (ADLs).

Observe increased forgetfulness with short-term memory.

 Watch for continuous and repeated questions to answers already given.

 Notice signs of confusion, impulsiveness, disorientation and unusual behavioral changes.

 Consult a physician who specializes in eldercare for a complete assessment.

 Follow-up with a family plan of action for care, which includes the older adult.

 Hire an eldercare consultant to complete an advance care plan.

 Assess the home for safety.

 Determine the need for healthcare aide services.

 Review insurance, trust and will documents.

CHAPTER 9

Elder Abuse: It Happened to Me

E lder abuse is the mistreatment of an older person that results in harm, injury or loss. Many would like to believe that this type of abuse happens only at the hands of people outside the family. In reality, it is a negligent act by a caregiver, or any person, which causes harm to an elderly. Abuse of any form is demeaning, embarrassing, and should not be tolerated; but, in some cases it becomes a daily part of life.

Steve, an 81-year-old man, told me one day that abuse doesn't have start off like some other extreme physical cases do, but that mental and emotional abuse, and not taking care of oneself are all forms of abuse. As a former football player for the NFL, Steve repeatedly mentioned, "I never imagined in my wildest dreams that I would end up here. How could this have happened to someone like me?" Steve's story begins as Laura's health began to decline due to diabetes, and he felt that he needed assistance to care for her. His wife Laura had always been the helpful one, but he stepped in and cared for her until the day she passed away. Over the three years of care, Laura went from having only daily glucose checks to dialysis- within a year -as a result of an aggressive decline in her health. Steve lived alone for the next 15 years, and as far as he was concerned, sustained a decent household. Steve golfed with his friends, and kept an active mind by working with the local middle school football coaches. Even though these are all positive outcomes for a widower, Steve felt that it was best he move closer to the city where his children were able to visit more often. According to Steve, his knee injury on the golf course was the beginning of a long road ahead, leading to him ending up in the hospital malnourished, his home condemned, and his daughter under arrest for elder abuse.

At 77 years of age, during the third round of golf, he took a swing and felt a sudden tear in his knee. He was rushed to the hospital, where they discovered that he had torn the ACL in his left knee coupled with a fracture in his ankle. Since his insurance didn't offer the best coverage, Steve didn't have the option to stay in a rehab center for 10 months as doctors had suggested, so he returned home after only four weeks. His daughter, a recovering alcoholic, moved into the home and became responsible for his care. As a former athlete, Steve formulated a modified rehabilitation plan for himself – deciding to rest daily and climb two or three of his household steps a day, in order to increase his strength. "I had the best intentions for myself, but I was ruining the healing process", Steve said. Since his healing was slower than he expected, he became depressed and some days, didn't want to get up or move at all. His daughter felt that she needed to help her father more, so she limited her workdays from 8 a.m. until 2 p.m. in order to assist him. She made herself available to help her dad move around the house to help expedite the healing process. During a tense moment, Steve lashed out at his daughter and she decided to give up her sobriety and have a drink. During her relapse, she disappeared for three days. Upon her return, Steve recognized his fault in the matter and told his daughter that he would be willing to work with her to get clean, as long as she continued to help him with his rehabilitation. This arrangement was successful for about six months until he re-injured his knee and had to begin the healing process all over again. His limited mobility caused him to depend on his daughter more than ever, and due to their increased living expenses, she began working two jobs.

Steve spent most of his days alone since he couldn't golf any longer. His friends would try to visit, but their health was beginning to decline as well, and the group began to dissipate. His daughter prepared meals for him and left food for the day. Steve grew tired of her and the level of care she provided. Feeling unappreciated, his daughter began to lash out at him, leaving food in in higher cabinets so Steve was unable to fend for himself during the day. His hygiene habits were almost depleted, and he was limited to showering once a week on his daughter's off days. The home grew to be an unstable and unclean environment. Due to the lack of income, modifications, such as a handicap ramp for Steve and a wheelchair could not be purchased. Because of the falling stairs behind the house and the flooded basement, the home became moldy, and as a result, Steve developed a bad cough. As he looked backed on some of these moments, he stated, "I'm a six-foot tall man, and I couldn't stand long enough to unlock the cabinets for food, or walk out of the house." His daughter grew mean, and Steve began losing weight. He believed that his daughter was doing the best she could, but they needed money to solve their problems.

"I have to deal with the circumstances", Steve concluded. After three and a half years of mistreatment, Steve called 911 because he had fallen out of his chair and needed immediate assistance.

When emergency crews responded, they found Steve in some of the worse living conditions they had ever seen. He had lost 46 pounds. Fecal matter and food were in his bedroom along with locked kitchen cabinets that contained food. Steve had neglected himself by not reporting his current living conditions. His daughter was emotionally and mentally abusing him, and the home was in disrepair, not to mention its contents were submerged due to the amount of water in the basement.

Steve was sent to the hospital to receive proper nutrition and then moved to a rehab facility. After just six months, he was able to walk 15 steps for the first time in almost two years.

Steve says that no matter who you are you have to think for yourself. You cannot always depend on your children to do the right things for you. You have to prepare yourself for whatever life brings to your doorstep. He says that as a football player with golfing buddies, "I never prepared for my friends to pass away and I mentally deal with it. For my income to be so limited, I needed help from my daughter. She always had the best intentions and her main concern was to not lose the home her dad built, but instead she lost herself in the process." Steve is now an advocate for elder abuse awareness. He wants others to know that it can happen to anyone, and that sometimes, it begins in a subtle manner. As he heads out to his daughters hearing, his goal is for the judge to see things from his perspective. His daughter isn't a criminal, but guilty of making bad decisions and not focusing on human needs. Steve expresses his sentiment, saying: "If you find yourself asking how this could happen to you, ask what you could have done to prevent this?"

Preventing Elder Abuse

The American Psychological Association (APA) statistics show that for every abuse case reported, at least 23 cases go unreported. This is a social problem, and its consequences jeopardize the health and welfare of human lives. In some cases, those affected decide to give up on living. There is despair, hopelessness, pain, hunger, loneliness and trauma. None of these conditions add substance to life.

Abuse must be recognized as an act of violence. There are signs to look for and strategies for protecting elders. Let's examine the five types of abuse, the first being self-neglect. How can someone abuse him or herself? Interestingly, when older adults are left to care for themselves alone, abuse could be in the form of unclean living conditions, poor hygiene, and malnutrition. Taking medication incorrectly and food not properly stored is also considered a form of abuse. Many older adults have pets and are unable to clean up after them; therefore, urine and fecal matter become overbearing in the home. If the elders refuse help from others, isn't following proper safety precautions, and getting medical attention for fear of discovery of their living conditions, this is also considered abuse.

Which leads us to physical abuse, including, but not limited to, broken bones, bruises, burns and the use of restraints. Elders are often pushed around, prodded and poked. As older people age, many of their normal habits change: instead of shoes with laces, slip on or Velcro would be a safer alternative. Instead of eating out, most meals are made at home. Fewer outdoor activities and more diet changes. When the diet changes, sometimes the caregivers will force-feed: this is abuse!

Thirdly, there is financial abuse or exploitation. The older adult is subject to a depletion of funds to care for him or herself and to purchase necessary items. Often, abusers will write checks forging sig- natures, stealing credit cards, or other valuables. There is also a potential to have an unexplained transfer of assets, sudden appearance of family members who were not around during care, or overall sudden changes in spending.

The next form of abuse is emotional: being agitated or made to express an emotion such as anger, sadness, or frustration. Being yelled at or ignored. Older persons are often the subject of abusers hollering at them, name-calling, cursing and threatening.

Lastly, there is sexual abuse. There will be noticeable marks on the body or bruising. The genital area may be infected or bleeding. Abusers will show older adults pornography and engage in non-consensual sex.

One of most effective ways in preventing elder abuse is to be a good listener. Many elders will be able to hint at the abuse happening to them. Keep your eyes and ears open. Observe changes in the environment and behavior of your loved ones. If capable, the older adult will show signs of not wanting to be left alone with the abuser. Explain to the older adult that it's always OK to tell someone they trust about their concerns. Attempt to educate the older adult about inappropriate behavior and their right to no physical contact.

Key Takeaways:

 A family member, caregiver or stranger can inflict abuse on an older person.

 Listen to the older adult as he or she begins to tell you things that concern them.

 Watch for fears to be left alone with the potential abuser.

 Notice physical signs of bruising, bleeding or broken bones.

 If using outside sources, check for licensing, certifications, references and the abuse registry.

 Check the finances of the older adult often.

 Look for missing or moved valuables in the home.

 In the case of abuse, call the police to make a report. Get the abused to a hospital immediately.

 Contact Adult Protective Services.

 Contact Office of the Aging.

 Contact an attorney.

CHAPTER 10

Passing on the Lessons Learned

Understanding why traumatic events occur is not where the focus should be, but should consequently be on how you can learn from the experience and passing along the lessons learned. This was my duty when I met Franzillo Wright.

She was an exceptional woman: a homemaker and remarkable grandmother. One of my fondest first memories of her was around six years of age when I could barely reach the kitchen counter, and wanting to watch her gut a catfish. She had a sense of humor and sarcasm that everyone loved. She always dressed like a CEO; sporting two-piece suits from Sax Fifth Avenue and Neiman Marcus. Her weekly routines included trips to the market, a 3 p.m. walk to play lotto numbers, and the bus ride to the hair salon on Thursday's, so she could be ready for church. She explained her life in some of the simplest forms: not living outside of her means and following a daily routine. She only involved herself with a limited number of people and used resources in the community such as centers, or focus groups, to learn about new technology or events in her city.

Her nationality was Venezuelan. Her family had settled in North America in the late 1800's, and she was born in Cleveland, Ohio in 1924. She was infatuated with maps; her dream was to visit her parent's homelands of Caracas, Venezuela and Sydney, Australia. During her lifetime, she had traveled to every continent except for Australia and Antarctica, and once retired, she took yearly trips to Las Vegas with a group of girlfriends. As a homemaker, she occasionally looked after the neighborhood kids, made dresses, and attended church functions in between excursions.

As I grew old enough to understand her, I felt as though our connection evolved when she experienced the death of one of her close travel friends. I watched her behavior change and I began asking questions. At the tender age of 10, I would ask, "Do you feel alone?" A flood of feelings and information began to spark a heartfelt conversation. She explained that she had been married twice and only had one son. Her hilarious claim to fame was gaining 10 pounds during pregnancy, and delivering a seven-pound baby.

She loved her family and always longed for a daughter. Grandma took a young mother under her wings and helped to raise her three small daughters. "I'm not alone, but sometimes I get lonely when I think of my husband," she would say.

During her second marriage, she began planning for how she wanted to live her life. A few more years went by subsequently, making her reflect on her state of loneliness. I raised the question again when her sister passed away, and once more as another one of her friends passed. I prayed for answers and was given the life's lesson I now currently use.

She went on to tell how her husband was shot in the leg one afternoon leaving work, and his head hit the concrete with enough strength to cause a blunt force trauma to the skull. He was treated and released after a few weeks, and she took over his care. He returned to work several months later, but soon retired due to constant headaches preventing him from working comfortably. She said that caregiving is required of everyone, and should be treated as a serious duty no matter what the relationship is with the individual in need.

After the death of her husband, she decided to make a plan called APC (already planned care), and kept it stored in a small, locked box. When I was 13, she handed me the key. I wasn't fully aware of the contents, yet, I was told to open the box in the event she could no longer speak or do it for herself. She confessed that she was diagnosed with lupus and now needed to be on medication. Her doctors at Cleveland Clinic treated her with the leading medical technology available and she was able to manage her condition.

Her blood relatives took over the managing of her affairs and home. Needless to say, communication became turbulent between her blood relatives and my family. Eventually, the police, The Office of the Aging and Adult Protective Services were involved. Grandma dismissively mentioned that violence she experienced would pass, but always gave the reminder to not lose the key for her locked box.

One evening as I visited, a relative of hers met me at the door. I was told I could only visit my grandmother as the family allowed it. Shocked, I responded that I too was her family, but reality began to set in as I realized I was not a blood relative. It was difficult for my family, but we all respected the request. It became a constant battle and dispute to visit, and so Grandma began meeting me outside of the home. I asked her what she needed from me, and, for the last time, the reply was for me not to lose the key. I battled internally with understanding where this was headed, but in hindsight it was one of the most important exchanges between the two of us.

Franzillo's health, both mentally and physically, began to decline right before my eyes. One evening, I called the authorities asking for assistance to check-up on her. Allegations were difficult to prove, and in the presence of an officer, Grandma was questioned about the abuse but denied any acts of malice towards her. We made eye contact and she motioned the turning of a key with her hand. The next day, I told my parents about the key she'd given me.

The authorities were called to her home again, and this time I expressed my concern for her well being, and justifying how I felt we were related. So the police asked me to leave and I told them I would be back in the morning after everything settled. I wasn't allowed in the house until the next day. I was given the warning to be ready for an uphill battle. Later on that afternoon, I visited the Office of the Aging followed by Adult Protective Services. I was given a number of brochures and phone numbers of people I could contact for assistance. I left the office with intentions to get my grandmother to safety and to remove the abuser from her house.

During my quest, I returned to my grandmother's home armed with a camera in order to prove that she was being neglected and abused. I entered the home and found   perishable food items hidden in drawers, a disheveled bedroom, and a number of small insects. I asked what happened and she sobbed that she was afraid to go into the kitchen, for fear of being yelled at or pushed. She expressed that she was given lunch daily and a small dinner, but couldn't locate her checkbook to go buy food for the home. I gave her $10 cash and upon leaving the home was met by an angry family member. After being in the home, I asked if I could take her with me for a while. Her family agreed and gave me a time frame to return. I explained that I was only there to take her to the store and to grab a breath of fresh air. She expressed she wanted to leave and her family chose not to argue.

The day was spent at several doctor's offices and stores to give her a sense of normalcy, and as our date ended, she began trembling when we approached her home. She asked me how could I help, and whom would I contact if I were to make any changes. I told her about getting her to move into a home or with my family, but she was hesitant. She said if the plan were successful she would go along with it, however, if I were caught snooping around the house or seemed in any way devious to her family, she would deny that she needed to leave.

Two days after the outing, Grandma collapsed in her home from a heart attack and was rushed to the hospital. Upon getting this news, my family dashed to the hospital. I was met by a nurse and an assistant who explained that my family was not allowed to see her and under strict orders not to give us any information on her condition. Filled with anger, I found the social worker and case manager of the floor and stated my position, showing them photographic proof of my grandmother's abuse.

When I arrived at the back of the hospital unit, I passed her family in the hallway as they were leaving. I called them and explained that I only wanted to show my support and nothing else. We would not intervene in her care or ask for additional information. I also explained that we would leave the room when nursing staff came in to alleviate the pressure violating the request of privacy from the family. I pleaded that if anyone could visit to please allow myself, or my sisters to do so. Finally, there was a truce.

Grandma's condition needed to be monitored. She was transported to a nursing home where she lived out the remainder of her days. I told the family that she had her services planned and I had the key to the information. Her family suggested that they were doing what was in her best interest and they didn't want any assistance from me, or family. Thus, I never got a chance to use the key.

The Key Lesson

Eldercare has become a growing field around the globe and should be recognized as a vital stage within healthcare. Involving all parts of the family dynamic becomes increasingly important as older adults reach a place where they are unable to articulate needs, or final wishes. Having an advanced care plan with a team involved is the best way to address these issues. There are several steps to begin the process of caring for an older adult, and it involves more than just a physical or medical need. Care encompasses your legacy, final wishes, end of life plan, and legal documents expressing how you choose to live out your final days.

Open the conversation by asking how the elder would like to plan their legacy, record the response, and then bring it to the family. The next step is to talk through the care plan. Determine what the exact wishes are, and who should be involved with the planning. Follow-up with assessing the physical needs of the elder and determine if medical attention or housing placement is necessary. This should be a priority.

Older persons will often feel that they trying to appease multiple members of the family. When making end of life plans, some older adults use the opinions of family members to make everyone else happy instead of expressing what they want.

Provide the reassurance that what the older adult needs is most important. With the changes in family structure, compromising is the optimal option, however it may not be achieved. In today's society family dynamics include others who may not be blood relatives. Extended or blended families sometimes have to be included. Years of involvement and the acceptance of others as blood relatives can enhance the support unit. In this situation, you need to bring in or seek an elder care consulting company as a neutral party to facilitate the conversation.

In the case of Franzillo, a health event was the cause of her family settling the argument and deciding what was in her best interest. The question of was she safe in her home or was she being abused, was never answered. Do not let a health event or family crisis be the instrument that unites or destroys a family.

Do not be overwhelmed by the term "care", but more open to accepting that older adults around you need assistance, no matter the age or stage they are in.

Care for those whom you love and keep their best interest in mind. Make it Wright before it's too late.

Useful Resources

APPENDIX

Name	Government Office	Website	Phone Number
AARP		www.aarp.com	1888.687.2277
Boston Scientific		www.bostonscientific.com	1800.328.3881
Cleveland Clinic		http://my.clevelandclinic.org/	1800.223.2272
Legalzoom		www.legalzoom.com	1855.787.1922
Mayo Clinic		http://www.mayoclinic.org/	1489.301.800
National Association of Councils in Development Disabilities		www.nacdd.org	1202.506.5813
National Care Planning Council		http://longtermcarelink.net/	
National Funerals Directors Association		http://nfda.org/	1800.228.6332
U.S. Administration	U.S. Administration on Aging, NCEA	http://www.ncea.aoa.gov/index.aspx	1.855.500.3537
U.S. Govt.	Medicaid	http://medicaid.gov/	1800.465.3203
U.S. Govt.	Medicare	https://www.medicare.gov/	1800.633.4227
U.S. Govt.	U.S. Department of Health & Human Services	http://www.hhs.gov/	
U.S. Govt.	Centers for Medicare Medicaid	https://www.cms.gov/	
U.S. Department of Health & Human Services.	National Institute on Aging	https://www.nia.nih.gov/	
National Center on Caregiving.	Family Caregiver Alliance	https://caregiver.org/	
The National Academy of Elder Law Attorneys	The National Academy of Elder Law Attorneys, Inc. (NAELA)	https://www.naela.org/	703-942-5711

U.S. Department of Health & Human Services	Alzheimers.gov	http://alzheimers.gov/	1800.272.3900

APPENDIX B

State	Office of Aging Website	Elder Abuse Hotline Website	Elder Abuse Hotline Number
Alabama	Department of Senior Services	http://dhr.alabama.gov/services/Adult_Protective_Services/Adult_Protective_Services.aspx	1.800.458.7214
Alaska	Alaska Commission on Aging	www.hss.state.ak.us/dsds/aps.htm	1.800.478.9996 or 907.269.3666
Arizona	Arizona Adult Protective Services (APS)	https://www.azdes.gov/daas/aps/	1.877.767.2385
Arkansas	Arkansas Adult Protective Services (APS)	http://www.aradultprotection.com/	1.800.332.4443
California	Department of Aging	http://www.cdss.ca.gov/agedblinddisabled/PG1298.htm	1.800.231.4024
Colorado	Colorado Department of Human Services (CDHS)	http://www.colorado.gov/cs/Satellite/CDHS-Main/CBON/1251575083520	1.800.752.6200
Connecticut	Connecticut Department of Social Services	http://www.ct.gov/dss/site/default.asp	1.888.385.4225 or 1.860.424.5241
Delaware	Delaware Adult Protective Service (APS) Program	http://www.dhss.delaware.gov/dhss/dsaapd/aps.html	1.800.223.9074
D.C.	D.C. Department of Human Services	http://dhs.dc.gov/service/adult-protective-services	202.541.3950
Florida	Department of Elder Affairs	http://www.myflfamilies.com/service-programs/adult-protective-services	1.800.962.2873
Georgia	Division of Aging Services	http://aging.dhs.georgia.gov/	1.888.774.0152

waii	Adult Protective and Community Services Branch (APCSB)	http://humanservices.hawaii.gov/ssd/home/adult-services/	808.832.5115 (Oahu), 808.243.5151 (Maui, Molokai, and Lanai), 808.241.3432 (Kauai), 808.933.8820 (East Hawaii), 808.327.6280 (West Hawaii)
ho	Idaho Commission on Aging	http://www.aging.idaho.gov/	1.877.471.2777
nois	Department on Aging	http://www.illinois.gov/aging/Pages/default.aspx	1.800.252.8966
liana		http://www.in.gov/fssa/2329.htm	1.800.992.6978
va	Department of Elder Affairs	http://dhs.iowa.gov/dependent_adult_abuse	1.800.362.2178
nsas	Office of Aging Services	http://www.dcf.ks.gov/services/PPS/Pages/APS/AdultProtectiveServices.aspx	1.800.922.5330
ntucky	Adult Protective and General Adult Services	http://chfs.ky.gov/dcbs/dpp/adult+protective+and+general+adult+services.htm	1.800.752.6200
uisiana	Office of Aging and Adult Services	http://new.dhh.louisiana.gov/index.cfm/page/120/n/126	225.342.9722
ine	Department of Health and Human Services	http://www.maine.gov/dhhs/elderly.shtml	1.800.624.8404
ryland	Department of Aging	http://www.dhr.state.md.us/blog/?page_id=4531	1.800.917.7383
ssachusetts	Executive Office of Elder Affairs	http://www.mass.gov/elders/	1.800.922.2275
chigan	Office of Services to the Aging: MiSeniors.net	http://www.michigan.gov/dhs/0,1607,7-124-5452_7119-15663--,00.html	1.800.882.6006
nnesota	Minnesota Board on Aging	http://www.dhs.state.mn.us/main/idcplg?IdcService=GET_DYNAMIC_CONVERSION&RevisionSelectionMethod=LatestReleased&dDocName=id_005710	1.800.333.24.33

Mississippi	Mississippi Department of Health and Human Services	http://www.mdhs.state.ms.us/programs-and-services-for-seniors/adult-protective-services/	1.800.222.8000
Missouri	The Missouri Department of Health and Senior Services (DHSS)	http://health.mo.gov/safety/abuse/	1.800.392.0210
Montana	Montana Adult Protective Services	http://dphhs.mt.gov/SLTC/APS.aspx	1.800.551.3191
Nebraska	Department on Aging	http://dhhs.ne.gov/medicaid/Aging/Pages/AgingHome.aspx	1.800.652.1999
Nevada	Nevada, Aging and Disability Services Division	http://adsd.nv.gov/Programs/Seniors/EPS/EPS_Prog/	1.800.992.5757
New Hampshire	Department of health and human services	http://www.dhhs.nh.gov/dcbcs/beas/adultprotection.htm	1.800.351.1888
New Jersey	The Division of Aging Services	http://www.state.nj.us/humanservices/doas/services/aps/	1.800..792.8820
New Mexico	New Mexico Aging and Long-Term Services Department	http://www.nmaging.state.nm.us/Adult_ProtectiveServices.aspx	1.800.797.3260
New York	The New York State Office of Children and Family Services	http://ocfs.ny.gov/main/psa/Default.asp	1.800.342.3009
North Carolina	North Carolina Department of Justice	http://www.ncdoj.gov/Help-for-Victims/Elder-Abuse-Victims.aspx	1.800.662.7030
North Dakota	N.D. Department of Human Services	http://www.nd.gov/humanservices/services/adultsaging/vulnerable.html	1.800.451.8693
Ohio	Ohio Department of Job & Family Services	http://www.ohiolegalservices.org/public/legal_problem/domestic-violence/copy_of_adult-protective-services/qandact_view	1.800.342.0533
Oklahoma	Adult Protective Services	http://www.okdhs.org/programsandservices/aps/	1.800.522.3511

egon	Oregon department of Human Services	http://www.oregon.gov/dhs/spwpd/pag es/offices.aspx	1.800.232.3020
nnsylvania	Department of Aging	http://www.aging.pa.gov/Pages/default .aspx#.VeUGlflVhBc	1.800.490.8505
ode Island	Department of Elderly Affairs	http://www.dea.ri.gov/programs/protec tive_services.php	401.462.3000
uth rolina	South Carolina Adult Services	https://dss.sc.gov/content/customers/pr otection/aps/index.aspx	803.898.7318
uth Dakota	Advisory Council on Aging	http://dss.sd.gov/asa/services/adultprot ective.aspx	605.773.3656
nnessee	Commission on Aging and Disability	http://www.tennessee.gov/humanservic es/article/adult-protective-services	1.888.277.8366
xas	Texas Department of Family Protective Services	http://www.dfps.state.tx.us/Adult_Prot ection/	1.800.252.5400
ah	Utah Human Services	https://daas.utah.gov/adult-protective-services/	801.538.3910
rmont	Department of Aging and Disabilities	http://www.dlp.vermont.gov/protection	1.800.564.1612
rginia	Department for the Aging	http://www.valegalaid.org/issues/elder-law/elder-abuseadult-protective-services	1.888.832.3858
ashington	Aging and Adult Services Administration	https://www.dshs.wa.gov/altsa/home-and-community-services/adult-abuse-and-prevention	1.866.363.4276
est Virginia	West Virginia Bureau of Senior Services'	http://www.wvdhhr.org/bcf/children_a dult/aps/report.asp	1.800.352.6513
isconsin	Wisconsin Department of Health Services.	https://www.dhs.wisconsin.gov/aps/ind ex.htm	608.266.2536
yoming	Adult Protective Services	http://www.health.wyo.gov/aging/servi ces/AdultProtection.html	1.800.457.3659

Bibliography & References

Branson, A., & Dunkin, M. (2004). The caregiver's survival handbook: How to care for your aging parent without losing yourself. New York, N.Y.: Berkeley Pub. Group.

Beekman, S., & Musson, J. (2002). Eldercare 911: The caregiver's complete handbook for making decisions. Amherst, N.Y.: Prometheus Books.

Beekman, S., & Musson, J. (2005). The eldercare 911 question and answer book. Amherst, NY: Prometheus Books.

Beekman, S., & Musson, J. (2008). Eldercare 911: The caregiver's complete handbook for making decisions (Revised ed.). Amherst, N.Y.: Prometheus Books.

Casarett, D. (2014). Shocked: Adventures in bringing back the recently dead. Penguin Group.

Davis, C. (2010). Start your own senior services business: Adult day-care, relocation service, home-care, transportation service, concierge, travel service and more (2nd ed.). Irvine, Calif.: Entrepreneur Press.

Emmott, H., & Emmott, D. (2013). Without regrets: A nurse's advice about aging and dying. HCE Enterprises LLC.

Focus on the family complete guide to caring for aging loved ones: The official book of the Focus on the Family Physicians Resource Council. (2002). Wheaton, Ill.: Tyndale House.

Henry, S., & Convery, A. (2006). The eldercare handbook: A difficult choices, compassionate solutions. New York: HarperCollins.

Kane, R., & Ouellette, J. (2011). The good caregiver: A one-of-a-kind compassionate resource for anyone caring for an aging loved one. New York: Avery.

Mace, N., & Rabins, P. (1999). The 36-hour day: A family guide to caring for persons with Alzheimer disease, related dementing illnesses, and memory loss in later life (3rd ed.). Baltimore: Johns Hopkins University Press.

Marchetta, A. (1989). Elder care a resource and referral guide. Boston: Health Action Forum of Greater Boston.

Meyer, M., & Derr, P. (2007). The comfort of home: A complete guide for caregivers (3rd ed.). Portland, Or.: CareTrust Publications;.

Molloy, W. (1998). Caring for your parents in their senior years: A guide for grown-up children. Buff alo, N.Y.: Firefly Books.

Moody, H., & Sasser, J. (2015). Aging: Concepts and controversies (8th ed.). SAGE Publications.

Morris, V. (2014). How to care for aging parents: A one-step resource for all your medical, financial, housing, and emotional issues; foreword by Jennie Chin Hansen (Third ed., pp. 184-352). Workman Publishing Company.

Pierskalla, C. (2013). The best you can do: For yourself and your aging parent. Highland City, Fla.: Rainbow Books.

Puchta, C. (2004). The caregiver resource guide: Blessed are the caregivers (2004/2005 ed.). Loveland, OH: Aging America Resources.

Quan, K. (2009). The everything guide to caring for aging parents: Reassuring advice to help you support your loved ones. Avon, Mass.: Adams Media.

Rakich, J. (2004). Cases in health services management (4th ed.). Baltimore: Health Professions Press.

Rantz, M., & Stauffacher, M. (2009). How to find the best eldercare. Minneapolis, Minn.: Fairview Press.

Rhodes, L. (2012). The essential guide to caring for aging parents. New York, NY: Alpha.

Rosenblatt, C. (2015). The family guide to aging parents: Answers to your legal, financial, and healthcare questions. Sanger, California: Familius.

Satariano, W. (2006). Epidemiology of aging: An ecological approach. Sudbury, Mass.: Jones and Bartlett.

Taylor, D. (2006). The parent care conversation: Six strategies for transforming the emotional and financial future of your aging parents (Rev. and updated ed.). New York: Penguin Books.

Wickert, K., & Dresden, D. (n.d.). The sandwich generation's guide to eldercare.

You and your aging parents: Guide to legal, financial, and health care issues. (2009). New York: Random House Reference.

Notes